FROM MANAGING TO CONQUERING CHRONIC DISEASE

Expert Guide To Understanding, Overcoming, Chronic Diseases Causes, Recognizing Symptoms, And Pursuing Effective Treatments For A Life Of Optimal Health

DR. DASHIELL DANIEL

Introduction 7
Context & Purpose 8
Objective Of The Book 8
The Intended Audience 9
Synopsis Of Chronic Illnesses 10
Environmental Aspects Of Prolonged Illness 11
Influences From Genetics And Epigenetics 12
Behavioral Modifications 13
And Lifestyle Interventions 13
Advances In The Diagnosis And Treatment 14
Healthcare Systems And Public Health Strategies 15

CHAPTER ONE 18

UNDERSTANDING CHRONIC DISEASES 18

CHAPTER TWO 22

THE SIGNIFICANCE OF PROMPT IDENTIFICATION 22

CHAPTER THREE 28

EFFECTIVE MANAGEMENT STRATEGIES 28

CHAPTER FOUR 33

INTEGRATIVE APPROACHES TO TACKLE CHRONIC DISEASE 33
Holistic Medical Procedures 33
Mind-Body Link 34
Complementary Medicine 35
Individualized Medical Care 36
Models Of Collaborative Healthcare 37

CHAPTER FIVE   39

OVERCOMING PSYCHOLOGICAL DIFFICULTIES   39
CHRONIC ILLNESS AND MENTAL HEALTH   40
ESTABLISHING A NETWORK OF SUPPORT   42

CHAPTER SIX   45

MANAGING THE HEALTHCARE SYSTEM   45

CHAPTER SEVEN   50

PUBLIC HEALTH INITIATIVES AND PREVENTION   50

CHAPTER EIGHT   54

**TRIUMPHANT NARRATIVES AND MOTIVATIONAL
TRAVELOGUES**   54
TRUE STORIES OF OVERCOMING CHRONIC ILLNESS   55
KEY TAKEAWAYS AND LESSONS LEARNED   56
SUMMARY   57

In the field of public health and healthcare administration, the book "Chronic Disease" is extremely important. Offering an in-depth examination of numerous aspects associated with chronic illnesses, this book is an essential tool for medical professionals as well as the general public. An overview of chronic diseases, the objective of the book, the intended audience, and the motivation behind exploring their intricacies are all covered in the introduction section, which also offers a nuanced background.

In the first chapter, "Understanding Chronic Diseases," various medical problems are carefully defined, categorized, and the differences between acute and chronic illnesses are highlighted. Additionally, common types of chronic diseases are discussed. The reader's comprehension is enhanced by the examination of causes and risk factors, which include genetic influences, lifestyle decisions, and environmental effects.

The chapter establishes the groundwork for the next chapters by highlighting the significant impact that chronic illnesses have on quality of life.

In order to effectively manage chronic diseases, Chapter 2 emphasizes the value of early identification and prompt diagnosis. It explores a range of screening and diagnostic instruments, including genetic testing, imaging modalities, and blood tests, and it addresses the obstacles to early detection, including testing-related stigma and a lack of knowledge.

Chapter 3's main topic, "Effective Management Strategies," offers insights into various methods for controlling chronic illnesses.

Examining medication therapies, complementary and alternative therapies, and lifestyle adjustments like exercise, proper diet, and stress reduction are all included in this. The importance of patient empowerment and education in promoting efficient disease management is emphasized throughout the chapter.

In Chapter 4, "Integrative Approaches to Conquer Chronic Disease," integrative therapies and the mind-body link are emphasized as holistic health approaches are introduced. It examines the idea of collaborative healthcare models and personalized treatment, demonstrating a multifaceted strategy for treating chronic illnesses.

The following chapters include prevention tactics, negotiating the healthcare system, and psychological difficulties. A special emphasis is placed on patient advocacy, healthcare disparities, and community health initiatives. The book comes to a close in Chapter 8, which offers readers real-life experiences and insightful lessons by presenting the inspirational journeys and success stories of people who have overcome chronic illnesses.

In conclusion, "Chronic Disease" is a thorough and academically rigorous handbook that not only clarifies the complexities of chronic diseases but also provides helpful advice on how to prevent them, identify them early, and effectively manage them. For anyone looking for a comprehensive grasp of chronic diseases, researchers, policymakers, and healthcare professionals, this book is a priceless resource because of its distinctive format and in-depth analysis.

Introduction

With millions of victims and a heavy financial strain on healthcare systems, chronic illnesses have become a major global health concern. The rising incidence of maladies like diabetes, respiratory disorders, and cardiovascular diseases has made a thorough investigation of methods to combat these conditions necessary. The goal of this book is to explore the many facets of overcoming chronic illnesses by providing insights into the underlying mechanisms, preventative strategies, and cutting-edge treatments. The impetus for this project is the pressing need to tackle the epidemic of chronic illnesses and improve our comprehension of the intricate interactions of genetic, environmental, and lifestyle factors.

Context & Purpose

Chronic diseases have their origins in epidemiological transitions, which are characterized by the change in the primary causes of morbidity and mortality from infectious to chronic diseases. Examining the historical, social, and economic elements that have led to the rise of chronic illnesses as a global health emergency is necessary to comprehend this shift.

The great influence that chronic illnesses have on people's quality of life, productivity in society, and financial strain on healthcare systems motivates efforts to combat them. It is clear from examining the historical background and contemporary issues that a multidisciplinary approach is necessary for successful management, treatment, and prevention.

Objective Of The Book

This book aims to provide a thorough resource for academics, educators, policymakers, and healthcare professionals who want to learn more about chronic diseases. Through the provision of a comprehensive overview, evidence-based approaches, and recent research, the book seeks to equip interested parties with the necessary skills to devise and execute successful plans.

It also seeks to close the knowledge gap between science and real-world application by encouraging interdisciplinary cooperation in order to address the complex nature of chronic illnesses. The book aims to support current global efforts to lessen the burden of chronic illnesses through a holistic analysis.

The Intended Audience

This book is intended for a wide spectrum of people working in public health, research, and healthcare. Medical professionals, such as doctors, nurses, and allied health specialists, will gain important knowledge about the most recent diagnostic and treatment modalities. Scholars and researchers will gain from the thorough examination of underlying mechanisms and possible research topics.

The societal ramifications of chronic illnesses and evidence-based tactics for successful health policy will be more understood by policymakers. Teachers will discover useful materials for instructing and educating the upcoming generation of medical professionals.

Synopsis Of Chronic Illnesses

Examining the numerous ways that chronic diseases develop and affect different organ systems is necessary for a thorough knowledge of these conditions. Heart failure and coronary artery disease are two major types of cardiovascular disorders that make up the majority of chronic illnesses. Diabetes mellitus poses special prevention and management problems due to the complex interaction of hereditary and lifestyle factors. Asthma and chronic obstructive pulmonary disease (COPD) are two respiratory conditions that greatly increase the burden of chronic diseases worldwide.

The spectrum of chronic illnesses is further diversified by neurological diseases, musculoskeletal ailments, and chronic renal disease. This part of the book gives readers a general overview of the chapters that follow and a road map for navigating the complex network of chronic illnesses.

Environmental Aspects Of Prolonged Illness

Extensive research is necessary to fully understand the crucial role that environmental factors play in the development of chronic diseases. Chronic conditions are largely caused and exacerbated by environmental factors, which include air and water quality, pollution exposure, and occupational risks. The correlation between environmental factors and the incidence of chronic illnesses has been demonstrated by epidemiological research, highlighting the necessity of focused interventions.

An additional layer of complication is created by the way that climate change affects the intensity and spread of infectious diseases, which can lead to chronic health issues. This section highlights the significance of implementing sustainable practices for long-term health by critically examining the complex interaction between the environment and chronic diseases.

Influences From Genetics And Epigenetics

Determining the underlying genetic and epigenetic mechanisms of chronic illnesses is essential for targeted therapies and individualized medicine. Unprecedented insights into the genetic components of diseases like diabetes, cardiovascular disease, and some types of cancer have been made possible by advances in genomics. Similarly, a dynamic view of how environmental influences might impact genetic predispositions is provided by epigenetic alterations, which control gene expression without changing the underlying DNA sequence.

This section of the book explores the possibility for precision medicine techniques that customize interventions based on an individual's unique genetic and epigenetic profile. It does this by delving into the complex interactions between genetics, epigenetics, and chronic diseases.

Behavioral Modifications And Lifestyle Interventions

There is no denying the influence of lifestyle choices on chronic illnesses, and treatments aimed at altering behavior have great promise for both management and prevention. The risk of chronic illnesses can be either mitigated or increased by some critical variables, including dietary choices, physical activity, tobacco use, and sleep patterns. Evidence-based lifestyle therapies are discussed in this section; these include stress management techniques, food adjustments, and exercise regimens.

Technology integration is also looked at as a way to support long-term behavioral changes, including wearables and mobile health apps.

Through comprehension of the lifestyle-related modifiable risk factors, both consumers and healthcare providers can work together to develop long-term health solutions that work.

Advances In The Diagnosis And Treatment

The diagnosis and management of chronic diseases have been completely transformed by advances in medical technology and therapeutic techniques. Early detection and individualized treatment regimens are made possible by the transformation of the diagnostic landscape brought about by precision medicine, biomarker discovery, and innovative imaging techniques.

The development of tailored pharmacological interventions, gene therapies, and immunotherapies is at the forefront of the fight against chronic diseases. This section assesses the state of therapeutic and diagnostic advancements critically, emphasizing how they have the potential to change the paradigm for managing chronic diseases. It also looks at the difficulties and moral dilemmas that come with applying these innovative methods to therapeutic settings.

Healthcare Systems And Public Health Strategies

At the population level, combating chronic diseases requires a planned and coordinated strategy. In order to lessen the burden of chronic illnesses, public health strategies—which can include anything from policy initiatives and community participation to preventative measures and health promotion campaigns—are essential. Furthermore, a key component of the overall management of chronic diseases is how well healthcare systems function in terms of offering equitable, high-quality care that is accessible.

This section looks at effective public health initiatives, evaluates how healthcare policies affect the course of chronic diseases, and emphasizes the value of creating a cooperative healthcare ecosystem. This book attempts to address systemic issues in order to support the creation of strong public health plans and healthcare systems that are capable of successfully combating chronic illnesses.

the fight against chronic illnesses is a complex journey that involves a thorough comprehension of the underlying mechanisms, environmental variables, genetic and epigenetic factors, lifestyle factors, advancements in diagnostic technology, and public health initiatives. This book acts as a thorough manual, bringing together a variety of viewpoints to support educators, researchers, politicians, and healthcare professionals in their endeavors to alleviate the worldwide burden of chronic illnesses.

The book intends to contribute to the ongoing evolution of healthcare approaches that prioritize prevention, tailored interventions, and the well-being of individuals and communities by encouraging cross-disciplinary collaboration and encouraging evidence-based practices. It is critical to acknowledge our shared responsibility for creating a healthy future for future generations as we negotiate the complexity of chronic diseases.

CHAPTER ONE
UNDERSTANDING CHRONIC DISEASES

Chronic illnesses are a major burden on the world's healthcare systems, thus a thorough understanding of their origins, causes, and potential solutions is vital.

Definition and categorization: Chronic diseases are long-lasting medical problems that frequently last a lifetime. It's critical to distinguish between acute and chronic diseases.

Acute diseases manifest suddenly and usually go away quickly, whereas chronic diseases take longer to heal and require continuous care. Chronic diseases are divided into several groups by the World Health Organization (WHO), which includes, among other things, diabetes, cancer, chronic respiratory disorders, and cardiovascular diseases.

Different strategies for diagnosis, treatment, and prevention are needed for each group since they present different problems.

Causes and Risk Factors: Deciphering the intricate network of variables causing chronic illnesses is essential to successful treatment.

Genetic considerations are important since some people are born predisposed to particular illnesses. Determining susceptibility requires an understanding of how genetics and environmental factors interact. Lifestyle decisions including nutrition, exercise, and drug usage have a big influence on the onset of chronic diseases.

The prevalence of diseases like obesity and type 2 diabetes has increased due to the rise in sedentary lifestyles and bad eating habits. Environmental factors, such as exposure to poisons and pollutants, are part of the reason behind the rising worldwide burden of chronic diseases.

Impact on Quality of Life: Chronic illnesses have a significant financial impact on healthcare systems in addition to having a significant negative impact on the lives of those who suffer from them.

Patients frequently experience pain, psychological discomfort, and physical limitations, which can have a domino effect on social and economic issues. Increased healthcare costs and decreased productivity exacerbate the effects.

These illnesses are chronic in nature, requiring lifelong medical care, which puts a burden on patients and their support networks. Furthermore, the psychological consequences, such anxiety and sadness, highlight the necessity of holistic methods to managing chronic diseases that take into account both the mental and physical aspects of wellbeing.

creating successful plans for overcoming chronic illnesses requires a thorough grasp of these conditions. This knowledge includes describing and categorizing chronic illnesses, looking into the risk factors and causes of them, and realizing the significant influence they have on life quality. Innovations in medical, genetic, lifestyle, and environmental perspectives, together with interdisciplinary collaboration, are essential to addressing the growing worldwide burden of chronic diseases. We cannot expect to achieve meaningful progress in the fight against chronic illnesses and raise the standard of living for people and society everywhere unless we adopt a comprehensive and knowledgeable strategy.

CHAPTER TWO
THE SIGNIFICANCE OF PROMPT IDENTIFICATION

A key component of any comprehensive plan for efficient disease management and prevention, early detection is essential to the battle against chronic illnesses. It is impossible to overestimate the importance of early diagnosis since it enables prompt intervention, individualized treatment regimens, and better outcomes for those with chronic illnesses. Early detection not only increases the likelihood of a successful outcome but also lessens the strain on healthcare systems and raises patient satisfaction.

There are several reasons why early diagnosis is important. First of all, it makes it possible for medical practitioners to recognize illnesses when they may still be asymptomatic or only have mild symptoms. Early stages of many chronic disorders, like cancer and cardiovascular diseases, respond better to therapy, offering a window of opportunity to put therapeutic measures in place that can stop or slow down the progression of the disease. Furthermore, early detection makes it easier to put preventative measures and lifestyle interventions into practice, which lowers the risk factors linked to the emergence of chronic diseases.

The utilization of diverse screening and diagnostic instruments is crucial in attaining prompt detection. Finding biomarkers that point to underlying medical issues is made easier with the use of blood tests. These examinations can measure a number of factors, including blood sugar, cholesterol, and inflammatory markers, which can provide important information about a person's overall health. Imaging methods, including MRIs, CT scans, and X-rays, provide precise images of inside organs and can detect anomalies and early illness symptoms. Another effective approach is genetic testing, which identifies hereditary predispositions to specific chronic illnesses, allowing for individualized risk assessments and therapies.

A crucial part of early diagnosis are blood tests, which analyze a number of blood parameters to find anomalies or biomarkers linked to particular diseases. For instance, increased concentrations of a particular protein or enzyme may be a sign of underlying illnesses such renal or liver disease. Blood sugar monitoring is essential for the early diagnosis and treatment of diabetes, a chronic illness that affects many people worldwide. Blood tests are an essential tool for both targeted screenings and routine health check-ups due to their versatility.

Imaging methods such as CT scans, MRIs, and X-rays provide a non-invasive way to see into structures and spot anomalies. While MRIs and CT scans offer precise views of soft tissues and organs, X-rays are frequently utilized to diagnose disorders affecting bones and joints.

Treatment results can be greatly impacted by early tumor, blood vascular, or structural anomaly diagnosis. These imaging techniques are useful for tracking illness progression and therapy response over time, in addition to helping to diagnose existing disorders.

Genetic testing is a cutting-edge method that has transformed personalized therapy and early detection. Healthcare practitioners can detect particular gene mutations or variants linked to an elevated risk of certain chronic diseases by studying an individual's genetic composition. Personalized treatment plans, early interventions, and focused preventive actions are made possible by this information. Genetic testing is especially important for disorders like some cancers and inherited cardiovascular diseases that have a high genetic component.

Even though early detection has many advantages, there are a number of obstacles preventing its broad use. Lack of information among the general public and healthcare professionals is one of the biggest problems. Inadequate awareness on the significance of routine screenings and the accessibility of diagnostic instruments may result in postponed diagnosis and lost chances for prompt intervention. In order to overcome this obstacle, public health campaigns and healthcare education programs that highlight the value of proactive health management and regular screenings are crucial.

Another major obstacle to early detection is the stigma attached to testing. There are civilizations where people are reluctant to have screening tests because they fear negative social consequences, including discrimination, or the stigma associated with particular illnesses. Destigmatizing chronic illnesses and promoting a culture that values and emphasizes preventative healthcare are both necessary to overcome this barrier. Campaigns for education and awareness can be quite effective in busting myths and lowering the stigma attached to early detection initiatives.

it is impossible to exaggerate the significance of early detection in the fight against chronic illnesses. It is an essential component of efficient illness management and has several advantages, such as better treatment results, lower medical expenses, and higher patient quality of life.

Early disease detection is important because it enables timely intervention and individualized treatment regimens. In order to achieve early detection, screening and diagnostic tools like genetic testing, imaging methods, and blood tests are essential. To optimize the impact of early detection initiatives globally, however, obstacles including lack of awareness and the stigma attached to testing need to be addressed through extensive education and awareness campaigns.

CHAPTER THREE
EFFECTIVE MANAGEMENT STRATEGIES

As a result of the complex nature of chronic diseases, effective management techniques are essential to their victory.

Pharmaceutical interventions stand out as a cornerstone among the many techniques. Progress in pharmaceutical research has resulted in the creation of pharmaceuticals that target particular pathways linked to chronic diseases, expanding the options for medications and treatments.

These drugs try to alter the underlying disease processes in addition to relieving symptoms. Healthcare professionals are able to customize medication regimens for each patient, maximizing effectiveness while avoiding adverse effects, by using evidence-based medicine and conducting thorough clinical studies.

Complementary and alternative medicine, or CAM, is an additional therapeutic approach for managing long-term conditions. These methods, which have their roots in conventional procedures, give patients who are looking for integrative and holistic care more options. Combining complementary and alternative medicine (CAM) with traditional treatment programs promotes a patient-centered approach that values cultural sensitivity and personal preferences. CAM techniques, which range from acupuncture to herbal supplements, provide a variety of approaches that, when employed carefully, can enhance conventional medical treatments and help create a more thorough and individualized treatment plan.

A key component of overcoming chronic diseases is changing one's lifestyle, which includes a variety of areas like stress reduction, exercise, and nutrition. Diet and nutrition are essential for reducing the effects of chronic illnesses. Individual diet regimens can be customized to control blood sugar, control weight, and address nutritional shortages.

Patients who get nutritional education are more equipped to make educated decisions and take an active role in their own health. Exercise and physical activity are also powerful strategies in the management of sickness.

In addition to strengthening cardiovascular health, structured exercise programs also promote general wellbeing and help prevent and treat chronic illnesses.

In the management of chronic diseases, stress management is a subtle but essential part of lifestyle adjustments. Numerous illnesses, such as autoimmune disorders and cardiovascular ailments, might worsen under long-term stress. Treatment programs that include stress-reduction strategies like cognitive-behavioral therapy and mindfulness meditation can significantly improve patient results. Since mental and physical health are intertwined, holistic therapies that manage stress have a substantial positive impact on the general health of people with chronic illnesses.

An essential component of effectively managing chronic diseases is patient empowerment and education. Giving patients information about their ailments, available treatments, and self-care techniques encourages them to take an active role in their healthcare process.

It is the responsibility of healthcare providers to ensure that information is communicated in a clear and comprehensible way so that patients feel comfortable asking questions and seeking clarification. Patients who feel empowered are more likely to follow their treatment regimens, alter their lifestyles, and participate in joint decision-making with their medical team, all of which enhance patient outcomes and quality of life.

overcoming chronic illnesses requires a thorough and coordinated strategy that takes into account lifestyle, education, and medicine.

Medical management is based on the prudent integration of complementary and alternative medicine with effective pharmacological therapies. Lifestyle changes that include exercise, stress reduction, and nutrition are effective methods for controlling and preventing disease.

Ultimately, a collaborative healthcare environment where people actively participate in their own well-being is fostered by patient education and empowerment. The healthcare community may work toward a society that is more empowered and resilient in the face of chronic diseases by adopting these comprehensive solutions.

CHAPTER FOUR
INTEGRATIVE APPROACHES TO TACKLE CHRONIC DISEASE

Chronic illnesses pose a serious threat to world health because of their protracted nature and frequently complicated causation. Healthcare practices must undergo a paradigm shift in order to effectively address these disorders.

Adopting integrative methods that prioritize customized treatment, collaborative healthcare models, and holistic health practices is one possible direction. We explore the nuances of each idea in detail in this extensive talk, outlining how they might help combat chronic illnesses.

Holistic Medical Procedures

Integrative approaches to managing chronic diseases are based on holistic health practices. These methods acknowledge how a person's physical, mental, emotional, and social well-being are all intertwined with one another. The holistic approach addresses the underlying causes of chronic diseases in addition to only treating their symptoms. Holistic health techniques embrace lifestyle adjustments such frequent exercise, dietary adjustments, and stress reduction in an effort to foster a healing environment.

Holistic health differs from standard medical models in that it places more of an emphasis on preventative care and the promotion of general well-being.

This approach provides a more comprehensive approach to treating chronic illnesses.

Mind-Body Link

The recognition of the mind-body connection is an essential element of holistic health approaches. This idea emphasizes how mental and emotional states have a reciprocal impact on physical health. For example, stress has been linked to the onset and aggravation of a number of chronic illnesses. Integrative methods use mind-body practices to reduce stress and enhance general wellbeing, such as yoga, meditation, and mindfulness. Studies indicate that these behaviors may have a beneficial effect on immunological response and inflammation, among other physiological processes. This emphasizes the possibility of mind-body therapies as supplements to traditional medical care.

Complementary Medicine

Therapies that integrate complementary and alternative medicine (CAM) with traditional treatment are essential in the field of integrative approaches. A wide range of treatments are included in integrative therapies, such as nutritional supplements, herbal medicine, chiropractic adjustments, and acupuncture. Although the origins of these modalities may lie outside of the conventional medical paradigm, their incorporation into treatment programs shows a more comprehensive understanding of healthcare. Research has demonstrated that a few integrative therapies can help people with chronic illnesses feel better, manage their symptoms better, and get better results from their treatments. The integration of specific integrative therapies with evidence-based conventional medicine constitutes a sophisticated strategy that tackles the complex nature of long-term medical conditions.

Individualized Medical Care

Personalized medicine is a novel approach to healthcare that customizes treatment programs based on an individual's unique genetic, environmental, and lifestyle characteristics.

It was made possible by advancements in genomics and molecular biology. Personalized medicine promises more accurate diagnosis and focused treatments when it comes to chronic illnesses. Predispositions to specific disorders can be found by genetic testing, opening the door to early interventions and individualized risk reduction plans.

Comprehending a person's reaction to particular drugs might also maximize therapeutic benefit while reducing side effects. Personalized medicine offers a more sophisticated and successful approach to managing chronic diseases, marking a paradigm shift from the one-size-fits-all approach in clinical practice.

Models Of Collaborative Healthcare

The intricacy of chronic illnesses demands a shift away from compartmentalized healthcare delivery towards more cooperative approaches. Integrative methods encourage multidisciplinary cooperation by uniting medical specialists from various specialties to create thorough and well-coordinated treatment plans. Beyond conventional medical professionals, this collaborative paradigm include psychologists, nutritionists, alternative and complementary healthcare providers, and other specialists.

Collaborative healthcare models strive to meet the various requirements of people with chronic illnesses by encouraging candid communication and group decision-making. This integrative, team-based approach recognizes the significance of addressing the complex components of managing chronic diseases and improves patient outcomes as well as the entire healthcare experience.

combating chronic illnesses necessitates a diverse and integrated strategy that includes integrative therapies, individualized medicine, holistic health practices, mental-body awareness, and collaborative healthcare models. Together, these ideas mark a paradigm shift in the care of chronic illnesses toward one that is more patient-centered, preventive, and all-encompassing. The potential of these integrative techniques to revolutionize healthcare and enhance the quality of life for those with chronic illnesses is becoming more and more apparent as research delves further into their complexities.

CHAPTER FIVE
OVERCOMING PSYCHOLOGICAL DIFFICULTIES

The fight against chronic illness is not limited to the physical domain; it also involves addressing the complex psychological terrain that people encounter after a protracted medical condition.

It takes a complex effort for people to cope with a chronic illness; they must manage emotional upheaval, existential reflection, and adaptive coping mechanisms. Chronic illness has a psychological cost that frequently takes the form of anxiety, sadness, and a generalized sense of hopelessness. Patients struggle with the psychological effects of their illnesses, thinking about how their identities may change and feeling the emotional fallout from having their lives changed by disease.

People participate in a dynamic process of adjustment and resilience when managing a chronic illness. This entails actively looking for methods to reclaim a sense of agency and control in addition to realizing and accepting the restrictions placed on by the illness.

There are many different types of coping mechanisms, such as problem-solving approaches, cognitive restructuring, and emotional control procedures. Health care providers are essential in helping patients through this process because they provide therapeutic interventions that enable people to adjust to and successfully manage the psychological difficulties that come with managing a chronic illness.

Chronic Illness And Mental Health

The complex interactions that exist between chronic illness and mental health highlight the necessity of a comprehensive approach to healthcare.

Mental health problems are essential parts of living with a chronic illness, not only comorbidities.

There is clear evidence of a two-way interaction between mental health and chronic illness: on the one hand, the physical effects of the condition can make mental health issues worse, and on the other hand, mental health issues can make it more difficult to manage the disease.

People who struggle with chronic diseases are more likely to experience anxiety and depression in particular, which leads to a complex web that requires specialized interventions.

Comprehending and managing mental health within the framework of chronic illness demands an all-encompassing healthcare approach.

This entails incorporating mental health screenings into standard medical examinations, encouraging candid communication between patients and healthcare professionals, and putting into practice evidence-based interventions like mindfulness-based practices, cognitive-behavioral therapy, and psychoeducation.

Understanding the psychosocial aspects of chronic illness improves overall well-being and quality of life for those managing a chronic health condition in addition to improving mental health outcomes.

Establishing A Network Of Support

One cannot emphasize how important a strong support network is to overcoming chronic illness. Creating and sustaining a network of support is essential to a patient's journey because it offers information, emotional support, and practical help. Together, friends, family, medical experts, and community services provide the scaffolding that supports people coping with the challenges of long-term sickness. With the purpose of building resilience and enabling a more positive trajectory in disease management, the support system acts as a buffer against the mental distress and social isolation that frequently accompany chronic illnesses.

Family dynamics are essential to the support system because they provide caregivers and loved ones with emotional support, practical help, and a feeling of stability during the upheaval that comes with a chronic disease. In order to create a collaborative approach to disease treatment, healthcare professionals—including doctors, nurses, and mental health practitioners—contribute their knowledge and direction. By offering empathy, a sense of community, and shared experiences, peer support groups and community organizations augment the existing support system.

defeating chronic illness requires overcoming psychological obstacles, attending to mental health issues, and creating a strong support network. This holistic approach acknowledges the strong relationship between psychological and physical health as well as the significant influence that mental health has on the course of chronic illness.

Through the use of these concepts, health care providers can customize interventions that extend beyond the management of symptoms, promoting resilience and enabling people to negotiate the challenging landscape of chronic illness with a feeling of agency and community.

CHAPTER SIX
MANAGING THE HEALTHCARE SYSTEM

Access to Care: Since it directly affects the prompt and appropriate administration of medical therapies, access to care is a critical component in the fight against chronic diseases. In this context, healthcare disparities—a subtype of access to care—present a serious obstacle.

These disparities, which are frequently associated with socioeconomic status, race, ethnicity, and geography, show up as variations in healthcare outcomes and quality among different demographic groups. A multimodal strategy that includes policy changes, expanded healthcare infrastructure, and educational programs to support equal access is needed to address healthcare inequities.

Healthcare Disparities: These are differences between various demographic groups in the quality of healthcare services received and the results of those treatments. Numerous factors, such as financial class, race, ethnicity, gender, and education, might contribute to these differences. Conquering chronic diseases requires an understanding of and commitment to reducing healthcare disparities, since these injustices can result in inadequate treatment, delayed diagnosis, and worse health outcomes for particular populations. Communities, healthcare professionals, and policymakers must work together to pinpoint and address the underlying problems that underlie these discrepancies.

Insurance and Financial Aspects: Access to care and the management of chronic illnesses are greatly influenced by the financial aspects of healthcare. Because people with chronic illnesses frequently have high medical costs, health insurance is essential to their treatment plan. It can be difficult to navigate the complicated world of insurance coverage and comprehend the financial ramifications, though. In order to effectively combat chronic diseases, policies that reduce the financial burden on individuals and families with chronic illnesses must be put in place, as well as initiatives to increase coverage and enhance health insurance literacy.

Patient Advocacy: Stressing the active participation of patients and their representatives in healthcare decision-making processes, patient advocacy is a crucial concept in the fight against chronic diseases. By giving people the voice to express their needs, interests, and concerns, advocacy makes sure that these viewpoints are taken into account when creating treatment plans. Furthermore, patient advocacy is essential for lowering stigma, increasing community support, and increasing knowledge about chronic illnesses. The prioritization of efforts that enhance patient advocacy and promote a collaborative healthcare environment is crucial in the fight against chronic diseases.

Communication with Healthcare Professionals: The management and victory over chronic illnesses depend heavily on the efficient exchange of information between patients and healthcare professionals. Accurate diagnosis, adherence to therapy, and the general success of healthcare initiatives are all facilitated by open and transparent communication. In order to ensure that patients feel comfortable sharing their symptoms, concerns, and treatment preferences, healthcare providers must communicate in a way that is both culturally sensitive and easily understood. Furthermore, encouraging cooperation between patients and medical professionals improves shared decision-making, which results in more individualized and successful chronic illness management plans.

overcoming chronic illnesses requires a thorough comprehension and application of fundamental ideas linked to negotiating the healthcare system. The cornerstones of effective chronic illness management are patient advocacy, insurance and financial concerns, healthcare inequities, access to care, and communication with healthcare professionals.

Together, communities, lawmakers, and medical professionals can address these ideas to build a healthcare system that is patient-centered, egalitarian, and supportive of the efficient prevention and management of chronic illnesses.

CHAPTER SEVEN
PUBLIC HEALTH INITIATIVES AND PREVENTION

In order to combat the complex nature of chronic diseases, prevention and public health initiatives are essential. They do this by focusing on societal and environmental factors in addition to individual behaviors that may be contributing to the disorders' prevalence. This all-encompassing strategy combines community health initiatives, legislative lobbying, and primary prevention tactics to reduce the global burden of chronic illness on people.

The cornerstone of any effort to tackle chronic diseases is primary prevention. Through the reduction of risk factors and the encouragement of healthy lifestyle choices, these programs seek to delay the onset of disease. Essential elements of primary prevention include changing one's lifestyle to include a balanced diet, regular exercise, abstinence from tobacco and excessive alcohol use, and so forth. Public health campaigns and educational initiatives also play a significant role in increasing awareness of the value of early identification and intervention. Primary prevention efforts aim to lower the overall prevalence of chronic diseases in communities by educating people and encouraging proactive health behaviors.

Programs for community health are essential to the all-encompassing strategy for overcoming chronic illnesses. The goal of these initiatives is to create a community that supports healthy lifestyle choices and guarantees access to preventative care. Community centers, educational institutions, and local health clinics work together to execute programs that target certain health needs within a variety of communities. Campaigns for immunization, community-based interventions, and screening programs for early risk factor identification all help to lower the prevalence of chronic illnesses. Additionally, community health initiatives frequently stress the significance of social determinants of health, recognizing the impact of socioeconomic variables on health outcomes and working to establish fair access to healthcare.

The policy and advocacy for the prevention of chronic diseases are fundamental elements of an all-encompassing public health plan.

Public policies have the power to influence elements like food accessibility, physical activity facilities, and tobacco laws, which can affect how people make decisions about their health.

The goal of advocacy initiatives is to increase public and policymaker understanding of the value of giving preventative actions top priority. Advocates help to create an atmosphere that is conducive to healthy living by influencing legislation and supporting evidence-based policies. Policy actions could include things like limiting the advertising of potentially harmful substances, imposing taxes on unhealthy products, and creating rules for school nutrition. Effective policies that address the underlying causes of chronic diseases and advance long-term health must be developed and implemented in concert with advocacy organizations, public health experts, and legislators.

combating chronic illnesses requires a multimodal strategy that includes primary prevention techniques, community health initiatives, and policy and advocacy work. Together, these initiatives target the more general socio-economic determinants of health, community dynamics, and individual habits to produce a thorough framework for illness prevention. By implementing evidence-based public health interventions and adhering to equity principles, nations can considerably lessen the prevalence of chronic illnesses and enhance the general health of their citizens.

CHAPTER EIGHT
TRIUMPHANT NARRATIVES AND MOTIVATIONAL TRAVELOGUES

When it comes to beating chronic illnesses, success stories and motivational journeys are essential for giving those who are battling long-term medical difficulties hope and inspiration. These stories, which highlight people who have not only survived but also triumphed over chronic illnesses, frequently represent the triumph of human resilience. These tales are sources of motivation because they show that, with perseverance and dedication to efficient treatment programs, recovery is not only possible but also attainable. Analyzing these success stories offers insightful information about the many methods people use to fight chronic illnesses, from medication to lifestyle changes. These stories also provide a deeper insight of the psychological and emotional aspects of the journey, highlighting the significance of mental toughness in the face of protracted health issues.

True Stories Of Overcoming Chronic Illness

Narratives of individuals who have overcome chronic illnesses provide a nuanced viewpoint on the complex process of managing and recovering from such illnesses. These narratives delve into the lived realities of people navigating the intricacies of chronic conditions, going beyond clinical descriptions and statistics. Analyzing the specifics of these stories enables a comprehensive understanding of the difficulty's patients encounter, how it affects their day-to-day existence, and the coping strategies they use. These experiences offer essential insights into the dynamic nature of chronic diseases and the varied techniques people employ to regain control over their health, from the first diagnosis to the many stages of therapy and recovery.

Moreover, the analysis of many real-life narratives makes it easier to spot recurring themes and patterns, which adds to a more thorough knowledge of successful strategies for overcoming chronic illnesses in a variety of medical settings and circumstances.

Key Takeaways And Lessons Learned

Developing successful preventative and intervention methods requires an examination of the insights and lessons gained from the experiences of those who have overcome chronic illnesses. These are life lessons that go beyond the therapeutic setting and cover a range of topics, such as lifestyle decisions, psychological fortitude, social support, and availability of treatment. Developing thorough and patient-centered methods for managing chronic diseases starts with analyzing the elements that lead to positive results. Furthermore, by comprehending the subtleties of these lessons, researchers, policymakers, and healthcare providers can customize interventions to meet the particular requirements and difficulties posed by various chronic diseases. Through the process of identifying the most important lessons from a variety of experiences, the medical community can improve treatment protocols, preventive measures, and support networks for people coping with the challenges associated with chronic illnesses.

SUMMARY

beating chronic illness necessitates a multipronged strategy that includes medication, lifestyle changes, and strong psychological support. Narratives of triumph and inspirational travels function as potent inducements, demonstrating that surmounting chronic illnesses is a feasible obstacle. Real-life stories illuminate the dynamic character of patients' journeys and offer a comprehensive perspective of the lived experiences of those coping with chronic illnesses. Healthcare practitioners can get important insights into successful approaches to managing chronic diseases by looking at these tales and then customizing therapies to meet the various needs of their patients. The development of holistic treatments that address the psychological, social, and environmental components that impact the course of chronic diseases in addition to their physical aspects is facilitated by the lessons learned and takeaways. The combination of success stories, firsthand experiences, and important lessons offers a road map for overcoming these difficult health obstacles in a more efficient and caring manner as we traverse the complicated terrain of chronic illnesses.